The A

Firm, Tone, and Tighten
Your Abs, Butt, and Core
By Dale L. Roberts
©2015

The ABC Workout Plan: Firm, Tone, and Tighten
Your Abs, Butt, and Core

August 18, 2015
ISBN-13: 978-1517451172
ISBN-10: 1517451175
onejackedmonkey.com

Featured photos and exercises from
"The 90-Day Home Workout Plan: A Total Body
Fitness Program for Weight Training, Cardio,
Core & Stretching"
March 29, 2015
onejackedmonkey.com
ISBN-13: 978-1508865704
ISBN-10: 1508865701
All photos courtesy of Kelli Rae Roberts, January
2015

Additional photos and exercises from
"The 3 Keys to Greater Health & Happiness: A
Beginner's Guide to Exercise, Diet & Mindset
(Second Edition, March 2015)"
First edition ISBN 978-1-4675-9582-7
Current ISBN-13: 978-1508783831
ISBN-10: 1508783837
All photos courtesy of Kelli Rae Roberts,
November 2013

Table of Contents

Introduction

If variety is the spice of life, then I have just added a little extra flavor your world. *The ABC Workout Plan* is a supplemental guide or a companion manual to my past two fitness publications (*The 3 Keys to Greater Health & Happiness* and the Amazon best-selling *The 90-Day Workout Plan*). The exercises, instructions, and pictures are exactly the same. However, I put a different spin on the workout plans.

I found that many people look to focus and target their training on specific areas of the body. A common concern or problem area that I address as a trainer is the "core." Some people are looking to tone, tighten and firm the core and other supportive areas to it (i.e. abs, butt). In *The 90-Day Workout Plan* (The 5 Components of the Workout - Component 4: Core) I discuss what makes up the core and its importance:

> The core, also known as the trunk, addresses the major muscles that move, support and stabilize your spine. [1] This includes the entire abdominal area from front wrapping all the way around to the back, then the small muscles along the spinal column. These muscles help you bend forward, stand up straight, bend backwards and sideways, twist, draw your stomach in and stabilize the spine during movement.

Is focused training or targeting muscle groups a successful method? In regards to targeting muscle groups for area-specific fat reduction, I wrote in *The 3 Keys to Greater Health & Happiness* (Chapter 2: Physical Fitness - Core Exercises):

> Here are a few things to remember before doing core exercises:
>
> **Fact #1**: Isolated movements are not going to get you targeted fat reduction. In fact, your body will determine what fat to burn and where to burn it.
>
> **Fact #2**: The abdominal muscles are small, therefore, are just small tools in your arsenal to create fat burn. If you wish to lose stubborn fat, the best movements are compound and integrated movements that require large muscles. Washboard abs are not created through 1,000 crunches per day, but through smart movements that incorporate more caloric expenditure and strict nutrition intake.
>
> **Fact #3**: Working your abdominal muscles all the way up, down and around can alleviate potential back problems, posture issues and digestive health.

Knowing that isolated movements will not

provide targeted fat reduction, *The ABC Workout Plan* is merely an aid in your fitness pursuits. Yes, you can target muscle groups and get excellent results. After all, when you shed all of your excess fat, you can then admire all the hard work you put into your abs, butt and core. However, this supplemental guide is not a lose-weight-quick fad or magic wand to spot reduce fat.

The workouts included in this book are a fun way to spice up your workouts and hit your favorite muscle groups. Pick out an exercise plan to spice up your workouts and enhance the other routines included in my previous publications. I hope you have as much fun doing these workouts as I did in developing them. When you apply these exercises consistently and diligently, you'll soon see remarkable results. Then, you can look down and around to admire the work you put into improving your abs, butt, and core. Enjoy and have fun!

How This Book Works

If you are relatively new to fitness, I would recommend using the workouts that incorporate all three elements of the abs, butt and core. That way worked muscle groups have time to recover between each exercise set. When you find some workouts becoming easier, you can advance on to the more advanced, targeted training such as:

- Abs and butt
- Abs and core
- Butt and core

Then, there are the more advanced standalone routines that individually address the abs, butt and core. If you want to get laser-focused on your training, these independent plans are an awesome enhancement to any routine.

Some workouts are a little shorter to accommodate busy schedules or to add at the end of a workout. Most of the workouts can be shortened by the number of sets performed for adjusting to what you are capable of handling.

For ease of use, the electronic copy has hyperlinks attached to every exercise in the book. If you are unfamiliar with a particular movement, you can click on the hyperlink to review the instructions.

Review the entire workout prior to performing the routine. A few exercises require equipment such as dumbbells, a dip/pull-up station or exercise mat. Most of the workouts require little equipment which makes these routines highly portable and appropriate for any place at any time.

Dig in!

Abs, Butt & Core #1: Bodyweight Workout

Time: 45 minutes

	Exercise	Time	Rest
1	Free Squats	50 seconds	10 seconds
2	Front & Back Bend	50 seconds	10 seconds
3	Cross Crunch	50 seconds	10 seconds
4	Forward Lunges	50 seconds	10 seconds
5	Hands Together Side Bend	50 seconds	10 seconds
6	Bicycles	50 seconds	10 seconds
7	Step Ups	50 seconds	10 seconds
8	Helicopter	50 seconds	10 seconds
9	Bicycle Cross Crunch	50 seconds	10 seconds
10	Split-Leg Squats - Left	50 seconds	10 seconds
11	Trunk Rotation	50 seconds	10 seconds
12	Russian Twist	50 seconds	10 seconds
13	Split-Leg Squats - Right	50 seconds	10 seconds
14	Bridge	50 seconds	10 seconds
15	Russian Twist with Bicycles	50 seconds	10 seconds

Repeat x2

Abs, Butt & Core #2: Dumbbell & Floor Work

Time: 45 minutes

	Exercise	Time	Rest	Sets
1	DB Sumo Squat	50 sec.	10 sec.	3
2	DB Trunk Twist	50 sec.	10 sec.	3
3	Reverse Crunch with Leg Extension	50 sec.	10 sec.	3
4	DB Transverse Lunge - Left	50 sec.	10 sec.	3
5	Knee Lift - Left	50 sec.	10 sec.	3
6	Bicycle Cross Crunch	50 sec.	10 sec.	3
7	DB Transverse Lunge - Right	50 sec.	10 sec.	3
8	Knee Lift - Right	50 sec.	10 sec.	3
9	Pumper	50 sec.	10 sec.	3
10	DB Step Up - Left	50 sec.	10 sec.	3
11	Superman	50 sec.	10 sec.	3
12	Window Wiper	50 sec.	10 sec.	3
13	DB Step Up - Right	50 sec.	10 sec.	3
14	Planks with Leg Lift	50 sec.	10 sec.	3
15	Coffin Sit Up	50 sec.	10 sec.	3

Abs, Butt & Core #3: Floor Work & Single Leg Work

Time: 45 minutes

	Exercise	Time	Rest
1	Reverse Crunch	50 seconds	10 seconds
2	Bridge	50 seconds	10 seconds
3	Split-Leg Squats - Left	50 seconds	10 seconds
4	Reverse Crunch with Leg Extension	50 seconds	10 seconds
5	Bridge with Heel Raise	50 seconds	10 seconds
6	Split-Leg Squats - Right	50 seconds	10 seconds
7	Reverse Crunch with Rotation	50 seconds	10 seconds
8	Single Leg Bridge - Left	50 seconds	10 seconds
9	DB Single Leg Squat - Left	50 seconds	10 seconds
10	Russian Twist	50 seconds	10 seconds
11	Single Leg Bridge - Right	50 seconds	10 seconds
12	DB Single Leg Squat - Left	50 seconds	10 seconds
13	Russian Twist with Bicycles	50 seconds	10 seconds
14	Superman	50 seconds	10 seconds
15	DB Walking Lunge	50 seconds	10 seconds

Repeat x2

Abs, Butt & Core #4: Intense Routine

Time: 40 minutes

	Exercise	Time	Rest
1	Free Squats	50 seconds	10 seconds
2	Walking Lunges	50 seconds	10 seconds
3	Front & Back Bend	50 seconds	10 seconds
4	Trunk Rotation	50 seconds	10 seconds
5	Crunch	50 seconds	10 seconds
6	Reverse Crunch	50 seconds	10 seconds
7	DB Squat	50 seconds	10 seconds
8	DB Walking Lunge	50 seconds	10 seconds
9	Hands Together Side Bend	50 seconds	10 seconds
10	Helicopter	50 seconds	10 seconds
11	Legs Up Cross Crunch	50 seconds	10 seconds
12	Leg Lift	50 seconds	10 seconds
13	DB Step Up	50 seconds	10 seconds
14	DB Single Leg Squat - Left	50 seconds	10 seconds
15	DB Single Leg Squat - Right	50 seconds	10 seconds
16	DB Trunk Twist	50 seconds	10 seconds
17	Knee Lift - Left	50 seconds	10 seconds
18	Knee Lift - Right	50 seconds	10 seconds
19	Supported Knee Lift	50 seconds	10 seconds
20	Hanging Toe-Ups	50 seconds	10 seconds

Repeat

Abs, Butt & Core #5: Less Intense Routine

Time: 36 minutes

	Exercise	Time	Rest
1	Cat & Dog	50 seconds	10 seconds
2	Quadrupeds	50 seconds	10 seconds
3	Planks with Leg Lift	50 seconds	10 seconds
4	Crunch	50 seconds	10 seconds
5	Bicycle Cross Crunch with Leg Hold	50 seconds	10 seconds
6	Russian Twist with Bicycles	50 seconds	10 seconds
7	DB Squat	50 seconds	10 seconds
8	DB Lunge	50 seconds	10 seconds
9	DB Step Up	50 seconds	10 seconds
10	Single Leg Bridge - Left	50 seconds	10 seconds
11	Single Leg Bridge - Right	50 seconds	10 seconds
12	Window Wiper	50 seconds	10 seconds
13	Side to Side Crunch	50 seconds	10 seconds
14	Floor Angel	50 seconds	10 seconds
15	Reverse Crunch with Rotation	50 seconds	10 seconds
16	Pump Lunge - Left	50 seconds	10 seconds
17	Pump Lunge - Right	50 seconds	10 seconds
18	DB Transverse Lunge	50 seconds	10 seconds

Repeat

Abs & Butt #1: Bodyweight Circuit

Time: 30 minutes

	Exercise	Time	Rest
1	Free Squats	50 seconds	10 seconds
2	Crunch	50 seconds	10 seconds
3	Forward Lunges	50 seconds	10 seconds
4	Reverse Crunch	50 seconds	10 seconds
5	Step Ups	50 seconds	10 seconds
6	Russian Twist	50 seconds	10 seconds
7	Side Lunge	50 seconds	10 seconds
8	Coffin Sit Up	50 seconds	10 seconds
9	Bridge	50 seconds	10 seconds
10	Bicycle Cross Crunch	50 seconds	10 seconds

Repeat x2

Abs & Butt #2: Dumbbell & Ab Work

Time: 30 minutes

	Exercise	Time	Rest	Sets
1	DB Walking Lunge	50 seconds	10 seconds	3
2	Supported Knee Lift	50 seconds	10 seconds	3
3	DB Step Up	50 seconds	10 seconds	3
4	Russian Twist with Bicycles	50 seconds	10 seconds	3
5	DB Single Leg Squat - Left	50 seconds	10 seconds	3
6	Supported Leg Lift	50 seconds	10 seconds	3
7	DB Single Leg Squat - Right	50 seconds	10 seconds	3
8	Pumper	50 seconds	10 seconds	3
9	Single Leg Bridge - Left	50 seconds	10 seconds	3
10	Single Leg Bridge - Right	50 seconds	10 seconds	3

Abs & Butt #3: Floor Work

Time: 30 minutes

	Exercise	Time	Rest	Sets
1	Bridge	50 seconds	10 seconds	3
2	Side to Side Crunch	50 seconds	10 seconds	3
3	Side-Lying Leg Lift - Left	50 seconds	10 seconds	3
4	Side-Lying Leg Lift - Right	50 seconds	10 seconds	3
5	Reverse Crunch with Leg Extension	50 seconds	10 seconds	3
6	Single Leg Bridge - Left	50 seconds	10 seconds	3
7	Single Leg Bridge - Right	50 seconds	10 seconds	3
8	Floor Angel	50 seconds	10 seconds	3
9	Lower Superman	50 seconds	10 seconds	3
10	Window Wiper with Legs Up	50 seconds	10 seconds	3

Abs & Core #1: Floor Work

Time: 30 minutes

	Exercise	Time	Rest
1	Bridge	50 seconds	10 seconds
2	Crunch	50 seconds	10 seconds
3	Cat & Dog	50 seconds	10 seconds
4	Planks	50 seconds	10 seconds
5	Russian Twist	50 seconds	10 seconds
6	Window Wiper	50 seconds	10 seconds
7	Side Planks - Left	50 seconds	10 seconds
8	Superman	50 seconds	10 seconds
9	Side Planks - Right	50 seconds	10 seconds
10	Jackknife	50 seconds	10 seconds

Repeat x2

Abs & Core #2: Standing Up & Floor Work Circuit

Time: 26 minutes

	Exercise	Time	Rest
1	Front & Back Bend	1 minute 50 seconds	10 seconds
2	Hands Together Side Bend	1 minute 50 seconds	10 seconds
3	Helicopter	1 minute 50 seconds	10 seconds
4	Knee Lift - Left	50 seconds	10 seconds
5	Knee Lift - Right	50 seconds	10 seconds
6	Supported Knee Lift	50 seconds	10 seconds
7	Jackknife	50 seconds	10 seconds
8	Side Crunch - Left	50 seconds	10 seconds
9	Side Crunch - Right	50 seconds	10 seconds
10	Planks	50 seconds	10 seconds

Repeat

Abs & Core #3: Floor Work Hit & Split

Time: 11 minutes

	Exercise	Time	Rest
1	Quadrupeds	1 minute 50 seconds	10 seconds
2	Planks	50 seconds	10 seconds
3	Jackknife	50 seconds	10 seconds
4	Russian Twist	50 seconds	10 seconds
5	Side Planks - Left	50 seconds	10 seconds
6	Side Crunch - Left	50 seconds	10 seconds
7	Side Planks - Right	50 seconds	10 seconds
8	Side Crunch - Right	50 seconds	10 seconds
9	Window Wiper with Legs Up	50 seconds	10 seconds
10	Hip Thrust	50 seconds	10 seconds

Butt & Core #1: Stand Up Circuit Workout

Time: 32 minutes

	Exercise	Time	Rest
1	Free Squats	1 minute 50 seconds	10 seconds
2	Front & Back Bend	1 minute 50 seconds	10 seconds
3	Forward Lunges	1 minute 50 seconds	10 seconds
4	Hands Together Side Bend	1 minute 50 seconds	10 seconds
5	Step Ups	1 minute 50 seconds	10 seconds
6	Helicopter	1 minute 50 seconds	10 seconds
7	Split-Leg Squats - Left	50 seconds	10 seconds
8	Knee Lift - Left	50 seconds	10 seconds
9	Split-Leg Squats - Right	50 seconds	10 seconds
10	Knee Lift - Right	50 seconds	10 seconds

Repeat

Butt & Core #2: Weight Training & Floor Work Circuit I

Time: 30 minutes

	Exercise	Time	Rest
1	DB Squat	50 seconds	10 seconds
2	Knee Lift - Left	50 seconds	10 seconds
3	DB Sumo Squat	50 seconds	10 seconds
4	Knee Lift - Right	50 seconds	10 seconds
5	DB Single Leg Squat -Left	50 seconds	10 seconds
6	DB Trunk Twist	50 seconds	10 seconds
7	DB Single Leg Squat -Right	50 seconds	10 seconds
8	Bridge	50 seconds	10 seconds
9	Window Wiper	50 seconds	10 seconds
10	Superman	50 seconds	10 seconds

Repeat x2

Butt & Core #3: Weight Training & Floor Work Circuit II

Time: 30 minutes

	Exercise	Time	Rest
1	DB Transverse Lunge - Left	50 seconds	10 seconds
2	DB Trunk Twist	50 seconds	10 seconds
3	DB Transverse Lunge - Right	50 seconds	10 seconds
4	DB Step Up	50 seconds	10 seconds
5	Side Bends - Left	50 seconds	10 seconds
6	DB Walking Lunge	50 seconds	10 seconds
7	Side Bends - Right	50 seconds	10 seconds
8	Single Leg Bridge - Left	50 seconds	10 seconds
9	Planks	50 seconds	10 seconds
10	Single Leg Bridge - Right	50 seconds	10 seconds

Repeat x2

Abs #1: Love Handle Buster

Time: 10 minutes

	Exercise	Time	Rest
1	Bicycles	50 seconds	10 seconds
2	Side to Side Crunch	50 seconds	10 seconds
3	Bicycle Cross Crunch	50 seconds	10 seconds
4	Side Crunch - Left	50 seconds	10 seconds
5	Bicycle Cross Crunch with Leg Hold	50 seconds	10 seconds
6	Side Crunch - Right	50 seconds	10 seconds
7	Cross Crunch	50 seconds	10 seconds
8	Window Wiper	50 seconds	10 seconds
9	Cross-Body Crunch	50 seconds	10 seconds
10	Window Wiper with Legs Up	50 seconds	10 seconds

Abs #2: Lower Ab Floor Work

Time: 10 Minutes

	Exercise	Time	Rest
1	Lying Leg Extension	50 seconds	10 seconds
2	Reverse Crunch	50 seconds	10 seconds
3	Russian Twist	50 seconds	10 seconds
4	Leg Lift	50 seconds	10 seconds
5	Cherry Picker	50 seconds	10 seconds
6	Flutter	50 seconds	10 seconds
7	Jackknife	50 seconds	10 seconds
8	Hip Thrust	50 seconds	10 seconds
9	Floor Angel	50 seconds	10 seconds
10	Coffin Sit Up	50 seconds	10 seconds

Abs #3: Total Abs Workout

Time: 12 minutes

	Exercise	Time	Rest
1	Crunch	50 seconds	10 seconds
2	Lying Leg Extension	50 seconds	10 seconds
3	Side to Side Crunch	50 seconds	10 seconds
4	Jackknife	50 seconds	10 seconds
5	Legs Up Crunch	50 seconds	10 seconds
6	Bicycle Cross Crunch	50 seconds	10 seconds
7	Side Crunch - Left	50 seconds	10 seconds
8	Side Crunch - Right	50 seconds	10 seconds
9	Russian Twist	50 seconds	10 seconds
10	Legs Up Cross Crunch	50 seconds	10 seconds
11	Reverse Crunch with Leg Extension	50 seconds	10 seconds
12	Cherry Picker	50 seconds	10 seconds

Butt #1: Circuit Workout

Time: Varies

	Exercise	Reps
1	Free Squats	50
2	Walking Lunges	30
3	Step Ups	30
4	Side Lunge	30
5	Bridge	50
6	Rest	2 minutes

Repeat circuit x2

Butt #2: Dumbbell Hit & Split

Time: 30 minutes

	Exercise	Time	Rest	Sets
1	DB Sumo Squat	50 seconds	10 seconds	5
2	DB Lunge	50 seconds	10 seconds	5
3	DB Single Leg Squat	50 seconds	10 seconds	5
4	DB Step Up	50 seconds	10 seconds	5
5	DB Transverse Lunge	50 seconds	10 seconds	5
6	DB Walking Lunge	50 seconds	10 seconds	5

Butt #3: Floor Work Circuit

Time: 23 minutes

	Exercise	Time	Rest
1	Bridge	1 minute 50 seconds	10 seconds
2	Side-Lying Leg Lift - Left	50 seconds	10 seconds
3	Single Leg Bridge - Right	50 seconds	10 seconds
4	Lower Superman	50 seconds	10 seconds
5	Side-Lying Leg Lift - Right	50 seconds	10 seconds
6	Single Leg Bridge - Left	50 seconds	10 seconds
7	Rest	1 minute	

Repeat circuit x2

Core #1: Stand Up Morning Workout

Time: 12 minutes

	Exercise	Time
1	Front & Back Bend	2 minutes
2	Side Bends - Left	1 minute
3	Side Bends - Right	1 minute
4	Helicopter	1 minute
5	Hands Together Side Bend	2 minutes
6	DB Trunk Twist	1 minute
7	Knee Lift - Left	1 minute
8	Knee Lift - Right	1 minute
9	Trunk Rotation - Left	1 minute
10	Trunk Rotation - Right	1 minute

Core #2: Floor Work (Down)

Time: 21 minutes

	Exercise	Time
1	Cat & Dog	1 minutes
2	Planks	1 minute
3	Quadrupeds	2 minutes
4	Side Planks - Left	30 seconds
5	Lower Superman	1 minute
6	Side Planks - Right	30 seconds
7	Superman	1 minute

Repeat x2

Core #3: Floor Work (Up)

Time: 18 minutes

	Exercise	Time
1	Bridge	1 minute
2	Window Wiper	1 minute
3	Bridge with Heel Raise	1 minute
4	Window Wiper with Legs Up	1 minute
5	Single Leg Bridge - Left	30 seconds
6	Side Planks - Left	30 seconds
7	Single Leg Bridge - Right	30 seconds
8	Side Planks - Right	30 seconds

Repeat x2

Glossary of Exercises

Abs Exercises

Bicycle Cross Crunch

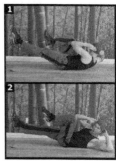

Lie flat on your back, support your head with your fingertips while keeping your elbows pulled back. Extend one leg 45° from the ground while drawing the other leg toward your chest. Simultaneously bring the opposite shoulder off the ground and drive that elbow toward the bent knee. Switch sides and repeat the movement sequence.

Bicycle Cross Crunch with Leg Hold

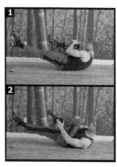

Lie on your back. Extend one leg 45° from the ground, draw the other leg into your chest and gently hug that knee while lifting the opposite shoulder. Release the hold and switch legs to repeat the movement sequence.

Bicycles

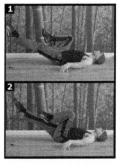

Lie flat on your back with your arms extended to your sides and palms faced down for support. Extend one leg 45° from the ground while drawing one knee toward your chest. Switch leg positions and alternate between legs for the entire exercise set.

Cherry Picker

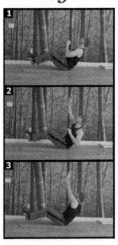

Come to a seated position on the ground with your knees bent and heels planted. Lean back onto your tailbone and reach your hands up. Reach higher with one arm then the other arm. Repeat this movement for the set.

Coffin Sit Up

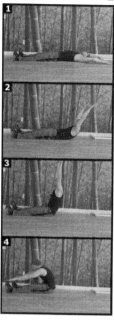

Lie on the floor with your arms by your ears, extended above your head. Slowly raise your back (one vertebra at a time) off the floor keeping your arms by your ears. When you have come to a seated position, reach toward your toes, pause, then slowly return to the start position.

Cross-Body Crunch

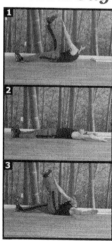

Lie on your back completely flattened out with your arms extended above your head. Simultaneously, raise one leg and the opposite arm up to the ceiling, lift your torso up to reach your toe. Pause, then slowly return to the lying position. Repeat the movement sequence on the other side.

Cross Crunch

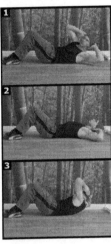

Lie on your back with your feet flat on the ground and your knees bent. Gently place your fingertips behind your head with your elbows pulled back. Slowly press one side of your ribs upward, pause at your highest position, then slowly return to the start position. Repeat the movement sequence on the other side.

Crunch

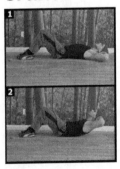

Lie flat on your back with your knees bent and your feet on the ground. Gently place your fingertips behind your head with your elbows pulled back. Slowly press your ribs upward, pause at your highest position, then slowly return to the start position.

Floor Angel

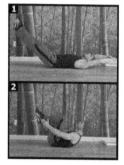

Lie on your back with your legs extended 45° from the ground and your arms raised above your head. Raise your upper body up as your draw your knees back toward your chest. Simultaneously sweep your arms outward and down to touch your ankles when the legs have come to meet the chest. Return to the start position.

Flutter

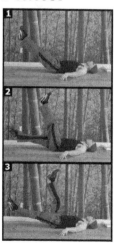

Lie on your back with your arms extended out to the side and palms faced down. Draw your legs together and up 45° from the floor (or higher for decreased difficulty). Move one leg higher than the other and alternate positions. Keep performing this sequence slow and steady while keeping your low back flat on the floor.

Hanging Leg Lift

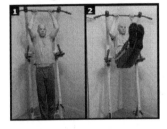 When you have mastered the knee lifts, you may progress to leg lifts by extending your legs to hip level. Breathe out as you lift your legs, pause, then tighten your midsection. Breathe in as you lower your legs back to the floor. Repeat this movement for a set number of repetitions.

Hanging Toe-Ups

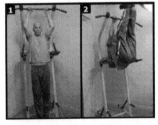 When you have mastered the hanging leg lifts, you may progress to toe-ups. This movement requires good flexibility in your legs for full range of motion. Begin by grabbing the bar with your arms extended overhead and a slight bend in your elbows. Your legs will begin extended below you. Breathe out as you collapse you extend your legs up to the bar you are holding onto. Pause, then tighten your midsection. Breathe in as you bring your legs back toward the floor. **<u>Caution</u>**: This is a tough advanced exercise and is not for beginners. If your grip is not good, you'll fall. Do not do this exercise if your legs are tight or inflexible.

Hip Thrust

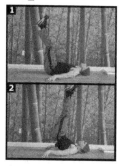

Lie on your back with your arms extended with palms faced down to aid in balance. Extend your legs toward the ceiling. Lift your butt and press your feet toward the ceiling, pause, then gradually lower yourself.

Jackknife

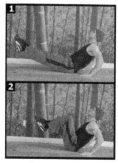

Come to a seated position on the ground with your knees bent and heels planted. Lean back onto your tailbone, extend your arms behind you with your palms placed into the ground for support. Extend your legs straight out, then draw your knees back in toward your chest. Repeat this movement sequence for the exercise set.

Leg Lift

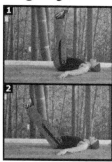

Lie on your back and extend your legs together 45° from the ground. Slowly raise your legs to point upward, then lower your legs to the start position. Repeat the movement sequence for the entire exercise set.

Legs Up Cross Crunch

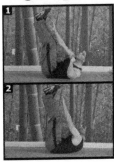

Lie on your back, extend your legs up and hold. Place your hands together, then slowly crunch up to reach one foot, pause at your highest position, then slowly return to the start position. Repeat this movement sequence in the other direction.

Legs Up Crunch

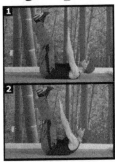

Lie on your back, extend your legs up and hold. Place your hands together, then slowly crunch up to reach your toes, pause at your highest position, then slowly return to the start position.

Lying Leg Extension

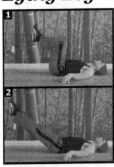

Lie on your back with your arms placed out to your sides and your palms down. Bend your hips, knees and ankles at 90° so that your lower legs are parallel with the ground and your low back is kept flat on the floor. Extend your legs out at 45° from the ground. Draw your legs back to the start position.

Pumper

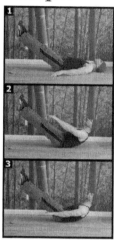

Lie on your back with your arms extended out to the side and palms faced down. Draw your legs together and up 45° from the floor (or higher for decreased difficulty) and lift your ribs up keeping your spine erect. Extend your arms along your sides parallel to the ground, then slowly pump them up and down for a timed set.

Reverse Crunch

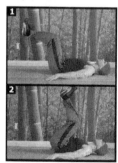

Lie on your back, place your arms out to your sides with your palms on the floor. Draw your legs to 90° bend at the hips, knees and ankles. Begin by lifting your butt off the ground and bringing your knees toward your head. Pause at the highest position you can, then lower your legs to the start position.

Reverse Crunch with Leg Extension

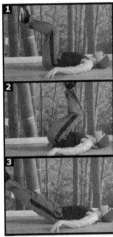

Lie on your back, place your arms out to your sides with your palms on the floor. Draw your legs to 90° bend at the hips, knees and ankles. Begin by lifting your butt off the ground and bringing your knees toward your head. Pause at the highest position you can, lower your legs to the start position, then extend your legs 45° from the ground. Return to the start position, then repeat the movement sequence.

Reverse Crunch with Rotation

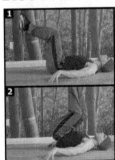

Lie on your back, place your arms out to your sides with your palms on the floor. Draw your legs to 90° bend at the hips, knees and ankles. Begin by lifting one side of your butt off the ground and bringing your knees toward your head. Pause at the highest position you can, then lower your legs to the start position. Repeat this movement sequence on the other side.

Russian Twist

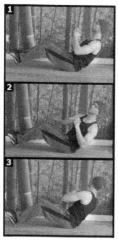

Come to a seated position on the ground with your knees bent and heels planted. Lean back onto your tailbone and clasp your hands in front of your sternum with your elbows bent. Rotate your torso to the left then to the right. Slowly repeat this movement sequence for the set.

Russian Twist with Bicycles

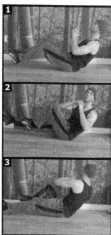

Come to a seated position on the ground with your knees bent and heels slightly lifted off the ground. Lean back onto your tailbone and clasp your hands in front of your sternum with your elbows bent. Rotate your torso to the left and bring your right knee up to meet your right elbow. Repeat this movement sequence in the opposite direction.

Side Crunch

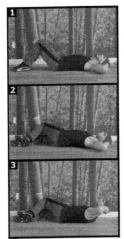

Lie on your back with your knees bent together and feet placed on the floor. Rotate your torso and bring both knees together to rest on the floor while keeping your shoulders flat on the ground. Place your fingertips behind your head and pull your elbows back. Press your ribs upward, pause, then lower yourself. Repeat the movement sequence for the entire exercise set and train each side equally.

Side to Side Crunch

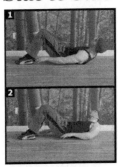

Lie on your back and place your feet flat on the ground with your knees bent. Press your ribs upward, pause at your highest position, then slowly reach with one arm to the same side heel and come back. Repeat the movement sequence as you reach to the other side.

Supported Knee Lift

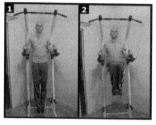

When you have mastered the traditional leg lifts, you may progress to a supported upright leg lift. However, I stress caution when choosing your piece of equipment. Begin with your arms extended at your sides, palms placed on your surface and posture upright in neutral alignment. Your legs will begin extended below you. Breathe out as you drive your knees upward. Pause, then tighten your midsection. Breathe in as you straighten your legs and extend them back to the floor.

Supported Leg Lift

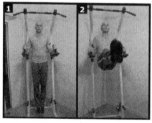

When you have mastered the knee lifts, you may progress to leg lifts by extending your legs to hip level. Breathe out as you lift your legs, pause, then tighten your midsection. Breathe in as you lower your legs back to the floor.

Window Wiper

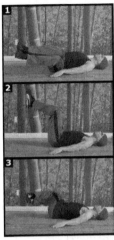

Lie on your back and place your extended arms to your sides for support. Begin with your legs bent 90° at the hips, knees and ankles. Slowly rotate at the torso toward one direction, bringing your knees together toward the ground. Squeeze your abdomen and draw your knees back to start position. Repeat the movement sequence in the other direction.

Window Wiper with Legs Up

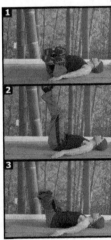

Lie on your back and place your extended arms to your sides for support. Begin with your legs straightened, pointing upward. Slowly rotate at the torso toward one direction, bringing your knees together toward the ground. Squeeze your abdomen and draw your knees back to start position. Repeat the movement sequence in the other direction.

Butt Exercises

Bridge

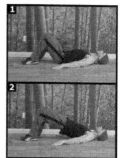

Lie on the ground with your arms out to the sides, knees bent and your feet placed flat on the floor. Press your pelvis up and hold when your torso is 45° from the floor. Pause, squeeze your butt and tighten your abs for a 3-count, then gradually lower your butt back to the ground. Repeat this movement sequence.

Bridge with Heel Raise

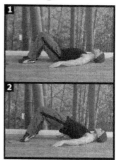

Lie on the ground with your arms out to the sides, knees bent and your feet placed flat on the floor. Press your pelvis up and hold when your torso is 45° from the floor. Raise your heels, squeeze your butt and tighten your abs for a 3-count, then gradually lower your heels and butt back to the ground. Repeat this movement sequence.

DB Lunge

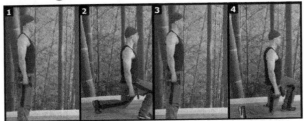

Grasp your weights at your hips and separate your feet shoulder-width apart. Step forward with one leg, bend at both knees. Pop up the rear heel and bring the knee close to the ground. Focus on a 90° bend in the front knee. Press your rear foot off the ground while driving your front heel down to bring yourself back to a standing position. Repeat the movement sequence on the other leg.

DB Single Leg Squat

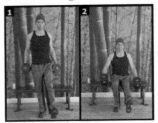

Sit down on a bench, extend one leg out in front of you and grasp your weights at your hips. Drive your other heel into the ground and stand up on that leg. Then slowly squat down on the same leg until you are seated again. If your balance is an issue, place the heel of your extended leg into the ground. After one set, switch sides to train equally.

DB Squat

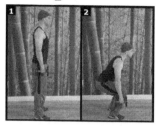

Grasp your weights at your hips with your legs shoulder-width apart. Come down to a seated position by bending 90° at your knees and butt. Press through your heels, keep your big toes lifted and extend your legs back up to stand.

DB Step Up

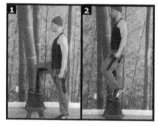

Grasp your weights at your hips. Place one foot on a bench and drive your weight through that heel to bring yourself to a standing position on the bench. At the same time as you start to step up, press off with the toes of your foot on the ground. When you come to a standing position on the bench, slowly lower the foot that pressed off the ground, then bring the driver leg to the ground. Repeat the movement sequence on the other leg to train equally.

DB Sumo Squat

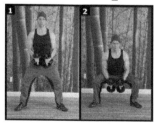

Grasp your weights at your hips and separate your feet wider than shoulder-width apart with your toes pointed outward. Bend at the knees and lower your butt as far as possible. Pause, then press through your heels and stand back up.

DB Transverse Lunge

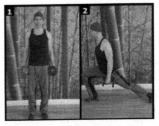 Grasp your weights at your hips and start with your feet together. Step one foot directly out to the side and turn your torso and toe outward before planting the foot. While keeping the other leg straight, squat down on the lead leg with a 90° bend in the hip and knee. Press off on the heel of your lead leg and come back to the start position.

DB Walking Lunge

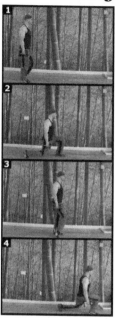

Grasp your weights at your hips and separate your feet shoulder-width apart. Step forward with one leg, bend at both knees. Pop up the rear heel and bring the knee close to the ground. Focus on a 90° bend in the front knee. Press your rear foot off the ground while driving your front heel down to bring yourself back to a standing position. Immediately bring the rear foot forward and begin the movement sequence on the other leg.

Free Squats

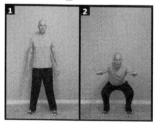

Place your hands at your hips with your legs shoulder-width apart. Come down to a seated position by bending 90° at your knees and butt. Press through your heels, keep your big toes lifted and extend your legs back up to stand.

Forward Lunges

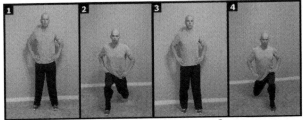

Place your hands on your hips and separate your feet shoulder-width apart. Step forward with one leg, bend at both knees. Pop up the rear heel and bring the knee close to the ground. Focus on a 90° bend in the front knee. Press your rear foot off the ground while driving your front heel down to bring yourself back to a standing position. Repeat the movement sequence on the other leg.

Lower Superman

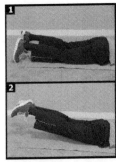

Lie flat on your stomach with your arms extended above your head, and palms placed flat on the ground. Your legs should be extended below you with your toes pointed away from your body. Squeeze your glutes for support and protection as you raise your hips from the floor. Keep both legs together as you aim to lift your thighs from the floor. Breathe out as you exert yourself to your highest position. Pause, then slowly lower your thighs to the floor while breathing in deeply.

Pump Lunge

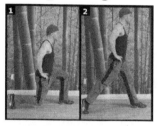

Separate your feet shoulder-width apart and place your hands on your hips. Step forward with one leg, bend at both knees. Pop up the rear heel and bring the knee close to the ground. Focus on a 90° bend in the front knee. Keep your feet in the same position and straighten both legs to a staggered standing position. Repeat the movement sequence for a timed set. Train both side equally.

Side Lunge

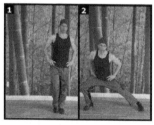

Start with your feet together and your arms loosely hanging at your sides. Step one foot to the side while keeping the other leg straight, squat down on the lead leg at a 90° bend in the hip and knee. Press off on the heel of your lead leg and come back to the start position.

Side-Lying Leg Lift

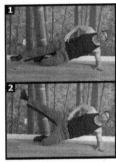 Lie on one side with your bottom knee bent and your top leg straightened. Place your bottom elbow into the ground with your forearm and palm placed flat to support and balance. Begin by lifting your top leg toward the ceiling while keeping your foot parallel to the ground. Lower that leg to the ground without touching, then repeat the movement sequence. Train each side equally.

Single Leg Bridge

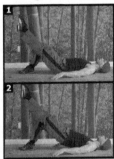 Lie on the ground with your arms out to the sides, knees bent and your feet placed flat on the floor. Extend one leg 45° from the ground. Begin by pressing your pelvis up and hold when your torso is 45° from the floor. Pause, squeeze your butt and tighten your abs for a 3-count, then gradually lower your butt back to the ground. Repeat this movement sequence and train each side equally.

Split Leg Squats

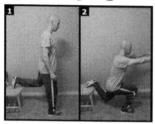

You need equipment, such as a chair or workout bench, that is sturdy and reliable for use in rear foot support. Place the equipment about 2 feet behind you. Extend one leg behind you with your toe placed onto the surface. You may need a wall, banister or secure surface for balance when first trying this exercise. Keep your front leg directly below your hip at the start with your posture in neutral alignment. The lead knee and hip will bend 90° and pause at the bottom. The further the lead leg descends, the more the back knee should slightly bend while the back hip extends. Slightly lift the big toe of the lead foot, drive your weight through the heel and extend the leg. When you press off the floor, tighten your midsection and breathe forcefully out, expelling all the air from your lungs. As you continue the upward movement, come to a full standing position with your lead leg returning to start position. When you are returning to this start position, carefully balance with the back leg. The feet should be forward facing and parallel at shoulder-width apart. Extend your arms at shoulder level when you squat down, then pull them back to your sides as you come up.

Step Ups

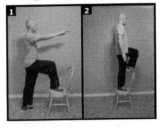

Precaution #1: Before beginning step ups, be sure to choose the item carefully that you will be stepping onto. It must be a steady and reliable surface to step onto with no obstructions or items nearby to trip or slip on. Please choose your item of stepping wisely and avoid using broken chairs or furniture that is less than safe to be stepping on. A sturdy chair with no wheels, a flat surface and braced against a wall is good for this exercise. Or more importantly, if you own a good workout bench or plyometrics box, this suits step ups best. Another option is using stairs or steps with hand rails for stabilization.

Precaution #2: After choosing the equipment for stepping up onto, be sure the work surface is not at a compromising height. Standing directly in front of your equipment, place one foot flat on the surface of your equipment. The knee should be lower than your hips. If your knee is higher than your hips, you must choose a lower work surface. It is detrimental to your knee to have it higher than your hip when you are stepping up.

With your equipment about one foot in front of you, place your leading foot flat onto the surface with your knee and hip bent no more than a 90° angle. Your back leg should remain straight with the foot planted. Your arms will begin extended directly in front of your shoulders. Press your weight through the leading foot while pushing off the floor with your back foot. Tighten the midsection as you forcefully exhale air out of the mouth. The lead leg will come to a full extension while having the back leg come up to tap the chair with the toes and keeping the knee slightly bent. During your ascent, use your extended arms for momentum by pulling them directly to your sides. Carefully return your back foot to the ground while bending the lead knee and hip to start position, no greater than a 90° angle. Breathe in deeply and have the back foot absorb the impact to return to the start position. Duplicate this motion and the same number of repetitions on both sides.

A couple options can be used in setting a good rhythm with step ups. One method is to keep your lead leg loaded up on the flat surface for the entire exercise, complete the set number of repetitions then switch to the opposite leg. The second method is to alternate legs with each step up. The latter method really builds great conditioning and endurance with a set rhythm.

Walking Lunges

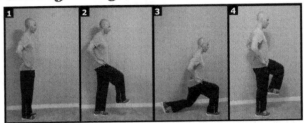

Place your hands at your hips and separate your feet shoulder-width apart. Step forward with one leg, bend at both knees. Pop up the rear heel and bring the knee close to the ground. Focus on a 90° bend in the front knee. Press your rear foot off the ground while driving your front heel down to bring yourself back to a standing position. Immediately bring the rear foot forward and begin the movement sequence on the other leg.

Core Exercises

Cat & Dog

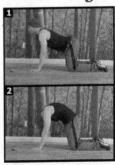

From a kneeling position and palms placed below your shoulders, arch your spine upward and look toward your knees. Then, push your spine downward and lift your chin upward.

DB Trunk Twist

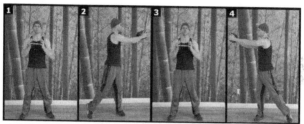

Grasp your weight in both hands in front of your sternum. Separate your feet shoulder-width apart and rotate your body to one direction. As you are rotating, extend your arms out toward that direction, then come back to the starting position. Repeat the movement sequence in the other direction.

Front & Back Bend

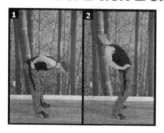

From a standing position, place your hands on your hips. Bend at the waist as far forward as you can go. Pause, squeeze your abs for a 3-count, then come back up. Without stopping, bend back as far as you can go, then immediately return to the start position.

Hands Together Side Bend

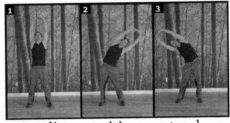

From a standing position, extend your arms overhead, interlace your fingers together and turn your palms upward with your biceps by your ears. Bend to one side as far as you can go and hold for a 5-count. Tighten your midsection and bring yourself back to the start position. Repeat the movement sequence on the other side.

Helicopter

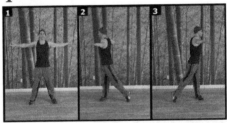

From a standing position, separate your feet shoulder-width apart and extend your arms directly outside your shoulders. Rotate at your torso, pop up the heel you are turning away from and pivot on the ball of that foot. When you have reached the farthest point, squeeze your abs, then return to the start position. Repeat the movement sequence in the other direction.

Knee Lift

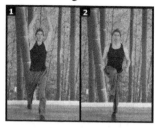

From a standing position, stagger your stance with your weight placed on the lead leg and the back heel raised. Draw your hands directly overhead and rapidly bring them down while bringing your rear knee up to meet in the middle. Quickly return to start position.

Planks

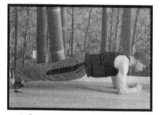

Begin with your legs separated shoulder-width apart and your toes placed into the ground for support. Place your forearms flat on the floor with your elbows bent at 90°. You should be straight from ankles to shoulders and keep your head at a neutral position with your eyesight set on your hands. As you hold your position, tighten your abs and butt.

Planks with Leg Lift

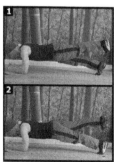

Begin with your legs separated shoulder-width apart and your toes placed into the ground for support. Place your forearms flat on the floor with your elbows bent at 90°. You should be straight from ankles to shoulders and keep your head in a neutral position with your eyesight set on your hands. As you hold your position, tighten your abs and butt. Then, lift one leg off the floor while holding your position steady. Alternate lifting a leg throughout the entire exercise set.

Quadrupeds

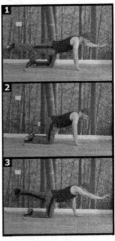

Come to a kneeling position, bend at the hips 90°, then place your hands below your shoulders with your arms extended. Raise one arm and the opposite leg parallel to the floor. Squeeze the butt and tighten the abs for a 3-count, then slowly lower back down. Repeat the movement sequence on the opposite side.

Side Bends

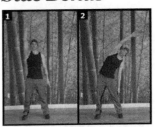

From a standing position, extend one arm directly overhead with your bicep by your ear. Keep your other arm directly at your side and bend your body directly to that side. Allow the downward arm to slide along the side of your thigh until your reach your full range of motion. Squeeze your midsection and bring your body upright.

Side Planks

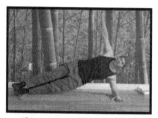

With your leg together, lie on one side with your left elbow bent 90° and forearm placed away from you onto the floor. Pop your hip up to the ceiling and point your free arm toward the ceiling. Keep your body straight from your ankles to your shoulders. After holding this position for a set, switch to the other side and train equally.

Single Leg Bridge

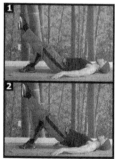

Lie on the ground with your arms out to the sides, knees bent and your feet placed flat on the floor. Extend one leg 45° from the ground. Begin by pressing your pelvis up and hold when your torso is 45° from the floor. Pause, squeeze your butt and tighten your abs for a 3-count, then gradually lower your butt back to the ground. Repeat this movement sequence and train each side equally.

Superman

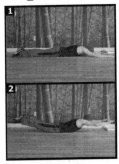

Lie flat on your stomach with your arms extended above your head. Lift your straightened arms and legs upward, pause then gradually lower them to the ground.

Trunk Rotation

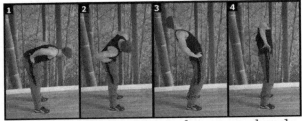

From a standing position, place your hands on your hips. Bend at the waist as far forward as you can go. Then slowly rotate from one side to the other.

Conclusion

Now that you have a whole new set of possibilities in your fitness pursuits get out there and use them. These tools will do you know good if you don't use them. Rest assured, these routines are tested and approved, so you will have no issue in getting remarkable results from using them.

Thank You

Thank you for taking the time to read my book. I hope that you enjoyed reading it as much as I enjoyed writing it. I have only one request; if you did like it, please leave a review. Reviews are the lifeblood of indie and small press authors and greatly help us get more books in front of more readers. If you didn't like it, that's fine too. Just leave an honest review, that's all I ask. Drop me a review on Amazon.com.

As you work toward your goals, you may have questions or run into some issues. I'd like to be able to help you, so let's connect. I don't charge for the assistance, so feel free to connect with me on the internet at:

DaleLRoberts.com
Like me on Facebook:
http://www.facebook.com/authordaleroberts
Follow me on Twitter:
@ptdaleroberts
Subscribe to my YouTube channel:
http://www.youtube.com/ptdalelroberts

Thank you, again! I hope to hear from you and wish you the best.
-Dale

P.S. My books are at Amazon Author Central at amazon.com/author/daleroberts. Click the "Follow" button to get updates any time I publish a new book.

About The Author

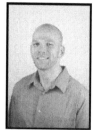

My name is Dale Lewis Roberts and I'm an American Council on Exercise Personal Trainer, Certified, with an ACE Specialty Certification in Senior Fitness. Since beginning my personal training career in 2006, I have earned numerous certifications in personal training, yoga, nutritional coaching, among others. I have worked with hundreds of clients with a variety of health & fitness goals.

While my greatest passions are health & fitness, writing and reading, I also love to spend time traveling with my wife, watching pro wrestling and playing guitar. I currently reside in Phoenix, Arizona, with my wife, Kelli, and our rescue cat, Izzie.

Subscribe to my blog at DaleLRoberts.com for all the latest posts on health and fitness tips. This is also one of the best ways to connect with me directly. Please, remember that whatever you do in life, make sure that you do what you love. Stay happy, healthy and strong!

Acknowledgements

My appreciation goes to my wife, Kelli, assistant, Carol Langkamp, and part-time editor, Colleen Schlea. And, my newfound focus on my health and fitness publications are due to Jason Bracht. He is an amazing mentor and friend. I really cannot thank all of you enough!

References

---

[1] Delaney, Bindi. (2013, October 11). Muscles of the Core. Retrieved from http://www.acefitness.org/blog/3562/muscles-of-the-core

Made in the USA
Middletown, DE
18 May 2017